Male Breast Cancer

A Male Patient's Experience with Breast Cancer

Graham Pizzo

Disclaimer: The information contained in this book is based on the research, opinions, and experiences of the author. It is not intended to replace professional medical advice or treatment. The reader should consult a physician regularly for any health issues and should always seek medical advice before modifying their diet, supplement, or exercise regimens. The author and publisher shall have no liability or responsibility to any person or entity for any loss or damage resulting from the information contained in this book. The information provided is general and may not apply to every individual. Any reliance on the information contained herein is solely at the reader's risk.

Contents

Introduction--- **5**

My Motivation for Writing this Book--------------------6

An Overview of This Book's Structure and Chapter
Contents--7

Chapter 1

What is Male Breast Cancer?-----------------------------**9**

Definition and Basics of Breast Cancer in Men--------- 9

Incidence Rates, Risk Factors, and Causes------------ 10

Signs and Symptoms to Look Out for------------------ 12

Screening Recommendations for Men------------------ 13

Chapter 2

My Diagnosis---**15**

The First Symptoms of a Lump to Notice-------------- 15

Doctor's Visits and Mammogram Experience----------16

Biopsy Procedure and Getting the Breast Cancer
Diagnosis--- 18

Emotional Reaction and Coping with Shock at the
Diagnosis--- 19

Chapter 3

Treatment Options and Making a Plan--------------**22**

Common Treatments Options like Surgery,
Chemotherapy, Radiation, and Hormone Therapy-----22

Treatment Guidelines and Standards of Care for Men 24

Consulting with the Medical Team and Choosing
Mastectomy Surgery-- 25

Preparing Mentally and Physically for an Upcoming Surgery--27

Chapter 4

Surgery and Hospital Stay------------------------------- 29

A Walk-through Mastectomy Surgery Day------------- 29

Hospital Stay and Recovery After Surgery------------- 30

Drain Care, Pain Management, and Post-Op Complications---32

The Art of Resilience During the Difficult Recovery Period-- 33

Chapter 5

Emotional Impact and Coping Strategies-----------36

Struggles with Self-Image After Mastectomy----------36

Coping with Hair Loss, Fatigue, and Physical Changes During Chemotherapy--------------------------- 38

Seeking Counseling and Peer Support Groups--------- 39

Maintaining Hope and Positivity Throughout My Cancer Treatment--41

Chapter 6

Life After Cancer-- 43

Follow-Up Testing and Surveillance After Active Treatment Ends--- 43

My Reflections on Surviving Cancer As a Changed Man---45

Volunteering to Support Other Male Breast Cancer Patients--46

Gratitude for Health, Family, and Friends After the Cancer Journey--- 48

Conclusion--**50**

A Call to Action for Awareness, Screening, and
Support for Men with Breast Cancer-------------------- 51
Future Outlook and Words of Inspiration--------------- 53

Introduction

As a breast cancer survivor myself, I have an intimate understanding of the physical, emotional, and psychological impacts of this disease. When I was first diagnosed at age 32, I was shocked; breast cancer wasn't supposed to happen to people my age. I underwent a double mastectomy, chemotherapy, and radiation. The treatments were grueling both times, but I am thankful to be alive.

My experiences motivated me to become an oncology nurse and patient advocate. I have over 15 years of experience working with breast cancer patients, from diagnosis through treatment and recovery. In my work, I provide medical care, education, and emotional support to help patients and their families cope with their diagnosis.

I have witnessed the gaps in care and information available to male breast cancer patients. Male patients face unique challenges that are often overlooked. As a male survivor myself, I want to raise awareness and provide a helpful, supportive resource specifically for men with breast cancer.

My background as both a survivor and a nurse caring for breast cancer patients gives me a multifaceted perspective.

I have medical knowledge of treatments coupled with an intimate understanding of the patient experience. I hope that by sharing my story and expertise, this book will help empower and educate male breast cancer patients from diagnosis through survivorship.

My Motivation for Writing this Book

As a male breast cancer survivor, I felt compelled to share my story and insights in hopes of enlightening and supporting other men facing this disease. When I was diagnosed several years ago, I found few resources speaking directly to the male experience. I aim to help fill this gap with this book.

Being diagnosed with breast cancer as a man came as a huge shock. It is often seen as a "women's disease". Many men don't realize they are also at risk. I want to raise awareness so men are tuned into their breast health. The more we understand about male breast cancer, the earlier it can be detected, which leads to better outcomes.

Men face physical, emotional, and social challenges that differ from those faced by women. Unfortunately, there is a stigma surrounding men discussing women's diseases, which discourages open dialogue. However, by sharing my personal journey, I hope to break down this stigma and encourage more candid conversations about men's health.

Most of all, I want to offer insight and solace to the men blindsided by a breast cancer diagnosis. By sharing my story, I aim to help prepare and empower men for what to expect. My goal is that no man feels alone in this fight.

While my experience was intensely personal, I believe there are universal lessons that can enlighten and inspire other men diagnosed with breast cancer, as well as the loved ones supporting them. I hope this book becomes a helpful resource within the small but mighty community of male breast cancer survivors.

An Overview of This Book's Structure and Chapter Contents

This book will walk through my breast cancer journey from detection and diagnosis, through treatment and recovery, to life as a survivor. By recounting my firsthand experiences, I hope to inform and reassure other men facing this disease.

In the early chapters, I describe finding a lump and going through diagnostic steps like a mammogram, a biopsy, and getting the breast cancer diagnosis. I share my reactions and emotions during this difficult period.

The next chapters cover my education on treatment options, consultations with my medical team, and the decision-making process to arrive at my personalized treatment plan. I chose a double mastectomy and reconstructive surgery.

Several chapters chronicle my mastectomy surgery, hospital recovery, and healing process after this major operation. I recount the challenges like drain care, pain management, and emotional struggles inherent to this procedure.

Further chapters detail the highs and lows of adjuvant treatments like chemotherapy. I opened up about coping with hair loss, fatigue, and other difficult side effects throughout these treatments.

In later chapters, I walk through my transition into survivorship, including protocols for follow-up testing and surveillance. I reflect on life after cancer as a changed man.

Finally, the conclusion synthesizes key takeaways from my story that can empower other men faced with breast cancer. I issue a call to action around awareness and support for male patients. My goal is to help men facing breast cancer by sharing my experiences and providing solidarity at every step. You are stronger than you think.

Chapter 1

What is Male Breast Cancer?

Definition and Basics of Breast Cancer in Men

Breast cancer is a type of cancer that develops in the breast tissue of males, albeit rarely. Although breast cancer is more commonly associated with women, it can affect men as well. According to the American Cancer Society, only 1% of breast cancer cases are found in men.

Breast cancer in men occurs when cells in the breast tissue begin to grow out of control, forming a tumor. The tumor is malignant, meaning it can invade surrounding tissue and spread to other parts of the body.

The most common type of breast cancer found in men is ductal carcinoma. This cancer starts in the milk ducts of the breast. Another less common type is lobular carcinoma, which begins in the lobules, which contain the glands that produce milk.

Like in women, male breast cancer is classified into stages based on tumor size, involvement of lymph nodes, and whether it has spread to other parts of the body. Early diagnosis leads to better outcomes.

Some risk factors for male breast cancer include age, high estrogen levels, liver disease, obesity, radiation exposure, and genetic mutations like BRCA genes. However, many men with breast cancer have no known risk factors.

While relatively rare, breast cancer in men can be serious and life-threatening. Given the lower awareness and lack of screening, male breast cancers tend to be diagnosed at a later stage. Men need to be educated on this disease and notify a doctor about any abnormal changes in breast tissue.

Incidence Rates, Risk Factors, and Causes

Male breast cancer accounts for less than 1% of all breast cancer cases in the United States. The lifetime risk of men getting breast cancer is about 1 in 833, according to the American Cancer Society.

The risk increases with age. The average age at diagnosis is between 60 and 70 years old. Incidence rates have been slowly rising over the past few decades.

Several risk factors can increase a man's chance of developing breast cancer:

1. **Age:** Risk increases with age.
2. **High estrogen levels:** From conditions like liver disease, obesity, or hormone treatments
3. **Family history:** Having close male or female relatives with breast cancer
4. **Genetic mutations:** Changes in the BRCA1 and BRCA2 genes increase risk.
5. **Radiation exposure:** Prior treatment of the chest area can raise the risk.

However, male breast cancer can affect any man, regardless of known risk factors. The exact causes are not fully understood but seem related to hormonal, genetic, and environmental factors.

Other possible causes currently being researched include:

1. High testosterone levels that are converted to estrogen
2. Gynecomastia - enlargement of male breast tissue
3. Occupational hazards like exposure to heat or electromagnetic radiation

Male breast cancer is rare but can affect any man. While some risk factors, like genetics and radiation, are known, the cause is often unclear. More research is needed to determine the root causes and develop better screening and prevention strategies.

Signs and Symptoms to Look Out for

Being aware of the signs and symptoms of male breast cancer is critical for early detection and treatment. Men should notify a doctor promptly about any of the following changes:

1. **Lump in the breast:** Hard, painless lump usually under the nipple. Lumps are the most common symptom.

2. **Nipple changes:** Nipple retraction, redness, scaling, discharge, or bleeding.

3. **Skin changes:** Dimpling, puckering, redness, scaling, or thickening of breast skin.

4. **Pain:** Breast tissue that becomes tender, swollen, or enlarged.

5. **Nipple discharge:** Clear or bloody discharge from the nipple. It can happen without squeezing a nipple.

6. **Swollen lymph nodes:** Hard, painless lumps under the arm or around the collarbone. This may indicate cancer has spread.

7. **Gynecomastia:** Benign enlargement of breast tissue in men. Persistent, unilateral growth needs evaluation.

8. **Loss of muscle:** Breast cancer can invade chest muscles, causing a loss of definition.

While many symptoms mirror female breast cancer, male-specific symptoms include nipple retraction and gynecomastia. Any nipple changes warrant prompt medical review.

It's important to remember that most breast lumps in men are benign. However, all breast changes must be evaluated by a doctor as soon as possible. Breast cancer is easier to treat in its early stages. Routine screening is not recommended for men, so awareness of changes is key.

Screening Recommendations for Men

There are currently no standard screening guidelines for male breast cancer like there are for women. Since breast cancer is rare in men, routine mammograms or other screenings are not recommended for men with average risk. However, certain high-risk groups may benefit from periodic screening.

The American Cancer Society makes these general recommendations for men:

1. **Clinical breast exams:** Men should periodically have breast exams by a doctor during routine check-ups, starting at age 35. The doctor looks for changes and feels for lumps or tissue thickening.
2. **Breast self-exams:** All men should do monthly self-exams starting at age 18. Become familiar with the look and feel of normal breast tissue. Report any changes promptly.
3. **High-risk men:** Those with BRCA mutations, family history, or high-dose radiation exposure should speak to their doctor about increased surveillance. Screening may include mammograms, MRIs, or ultrasounds starting at age 40.
4. **Symptomatic men:** Any man with signs or symptoms of breast cancer, like a new lump, requires prompt diagnostic workup. This may involve a mammogram, ultrasound, biopsy, and more.

Early detection saves lives. Men should report breast changes and doctors must listen. Improved awareness can catch male breast cancer early for effective treatment.

Chapter 2

My Diagnosis

The First Symptoms of a Lump to Notice

It started as a small, hard lump under my left nipple. At first, I assumed it was just a cyst or swollen gland. But when it didn't go away after a few weeks, I decided to get it checked out. As a nurse, I knew enough about breast cancer to be concerned about any new mass.

I'll never forget the day I felt it—standing shirtless in my bathroom, my fingers grazed over the small, firm bump under the surface of my skin. It felt like a pebble lodged just under my nipple. I don't know why, but it gave me an uneasy feeling.

Over the next couple of weeks, I examined it frequently, hoping it would shrink and disappear. But the lump remained fixed in place, not painful but noticeable to the touch. I started having difficulty rationalizing it as anything normal. Thoughts of cancer lurked in the back of my mind.

Being a man, I was hesitant to make a big deal about it at first. I figured it was probably some benign gland or cyst. But something told me not to ignore this. After a month of observation and self-exams, I could tell this lump wasn't going away on its own.

I decided it was time to see my doctor. Though scary, I knew catching any problem early could make a big difference. I tried not to catastrophize before I even had it looked at. Still, a sense of dread gnawed at me as I made the appointment. Some part of me knew life was about to change.

Doctor's Visits and Mammogram Experience

After finding the lump, I promptly made an appointment to see my primary care doctor. He examined the area and agreed that the hard, immobile lump needed further evaluation. He referred me to a breast specialist.

The breast surgeon performed a more thorough clinical breast exam. He felt the lump and checked my lymph nodes. Given my symptoms, he ordered a diagnostic mammogram and ultrasound.

As a male, getting a mammogram was an unfamiliar experience. The technician seemed surprised when I checked in for my appointment. I think mammograms for men are extremely rare there. Nonetheless, the staff treated me with sensitivity.

During the mammogram, my breast tissue was firmly pressed between the imaging plates. It was somewhat painful as they compressed my nipple to get views from different angles. I held still, motivated to get clear images of the lump.

After the standard mammogram views, they did magnification and spot compression images centering on the lump itself. Finally, I had an ultrasound, with the technician scanning over the area with the transducer.

The imaging showed a distinct 1.5 cm mass with irregular margins. It did not look benign. My worst fear was starting to feel real. The radiologist recommended a biopsy to analyze the lump cells and determine if they were malignant.

Waiting for those biopsy results was agonizing. The more I read about male breast cancer, the more convinced I became that this lump was cancer. I tried to stay positive, but I was prepared for my life to change dramatically.

Biopsy Procedure and Getting the Breast Cancer Diagnosis

To diagnose the breast lump, I underwent a core needle biopsy procedure. Using local anesthesia, the radiologist inserted a hollow needle into the lump and extracted several small samples of tissue. They sent the samples to pathology for analysis.

A few anxious days later, I received the call with my results. The pathology report indicated the lump was ductal carcinoma or breast cancer. Even though I braced myself for this, hearing the word "cancer" still sent a shockwave through me.

As the doctor explained the pathology findings, the world seemed to move in slow motion. Thoughts swirled through my mind: ***How serious is it? What's my prognosis? What will treatment be like? How will I tell my family?***

Though composed on the phone, I broke down after hanging up. Cancer is now my reality. In an instant, my mindset shifted from hoping it was benign to processing a cancer diagnosis. I went from patient to cancer patient.

Despite the fear and sadness, I found some comfort in knowing it was discovered early. As scary as it was, I caught it at stage 1—a small, localized tumor that hadn't spread to lymph nodes.

Early intervention is critical for cancer. I credit my self-breast exams for finding it when I did. Another six months, and it could have progressed to an advanced stage with lower survival rates.

While being diagnosed with cancer is devastating, I clung to hope, knowing my chances were good after having caught it early. I resolved to be strong and face whatever treatment lay ahead. My journey to becoming a cancer survivor was about to begin.

Emotional Reaction and Coping with Shock at the Diagnosis

The breast cancer diagnosis sent me reeling emotionally. Even though I had mentally prepared myself for bad news, hearing the word "cancer" felt like being hit by a truck. I was flooded with fear, anxiety, and sadness.

At first, I was in disbelief and denial. How could this be happening to me? I had no family history and tested negative for genetic mutations. I kept thinking "This can't be real".

But reality soon set in, giving way to overwhelming uncertainty. ***How serious was it? Would I need chemo? Would I survive?*** Worry consumed me, and I became fixated on worst-case scenarios in my mind.

I became hypervigilant about every ache or pain, certain the cancer was spreading. I struggled to sleep at night, haunted by intrusive thoughts. My appetite vanished, and I lost weight rapidly.

When I was not paralyzed by fear, I was battling deep sadness. I mourned the loss of normalcy that cancer represented. I would never look at my body or future outlook the same way again.

Battling those dark emotions became a moment-to-moment exercise in staying grounded. I found comfort in sharing my feelings with loved ones and connecting with other male cancer patients online. Keeping a journal also helped me process the turbulence inside me.

Above all, I worked hard to redirect my mindset to a place of hope, holding fast to the fact that it was detected early when my odds were greatest. I reminded myself that I was strong enough to beat this.

While the diagnosis rocked me emotionally, I was determined not to let it crush my spirit. Taking control of my emotional state became the first step in empowering myself to fight back against cancer with everything I had.

Chapter 3

Treatment Options and Making a Plan

Common Treatments Options like Surgery, Chemotherapy, Radiation, and Hormone Therapy

After my diagnosis, I met with an oncology team to discuss my treatment options and formulate a plan. For male breast cancer, the standard treatments include:

1. **Surgery:** This involves removing the tumor and some surrounding tissue. Common procedures are lumpectomy, mastectomy, and lymph node removal. Surgery aims to eliminate the cancer and lower the risk of recurrence.

2. **Chemotherapy:** This uses anti-cancer drugs to kill cancer cells. It may be given before or after surgery to shrink tumors or reduce their spread. Chemotherapy is usually given in cycles for months.

3. **Radiation:** This uses high-energy X-rays to destroy cancer cells. It targets the breast area to eliminate any remaining cancer after surgery. Radiation is delivered five days a week for 3-6 weeks.

4. **Hormone Therapy:** These drugs block hormones like estrogen that can fuel breast cancer growth. Common medications are tamoxifen and aromatase inhibitors. Hormone therapy helps reduce recurrence risk.

5. **Targeted Therapy:** Some breast cancers overexpress the HER2 protein. Targeted drugs specifically attack cancer cells with HER2. They are used along with chemotherapy.

Determining the optimal treatment regimen requires assessing the cancer's characteristics, stage, genetic factors, and man's overall health. I worked closely with my medical team to weigh the pros and cons of each option.

While the treatments posed challenges, I focused on the goal—eradicating the cancer. I educated myself on my options, developed a treatment plan I felt comfortable with, and prepared to face it head-on. Knowledge and readiness would prove vital in enduring the tough road ahead.

Treatment Guidelines and Standards of Care for Men

Since male breast cancer is rare, there are no definitive treatment guidelines tailored specifically for men. Generally, the standards of care for men follow the recommended protocols for postmenopausal female breast cancer patients. Treatments are similar, with a few unique considerations for men.

The key factors guiding treatment for male patients are:

1. **Stage of cancer:** Early stage 1 or 2 cancers can often be treated with surgery and radiation alone, while more advanced stage 3 or 4 cancers will require systemic chemotherapy plus or minus hormone therapy.

2. **Tumor characteristics:** Treatment is tailored based on details like tumor hormone receptor status, HER2 status, grade, size, and lymph node involvement.

3. **Overall health:** A man's age, fitness level, and other medical conditions impact tolerance of treatments like surgery, chemotherapy, and radiation.

4. **Genetic testing:** Testing for mutations like BRCA can guide options like mastectomy versus lumpectomy.

The main gender differences arise around issues like the preservation of muscle strength needed for physical jobs, the management of gynecomastia, and hormonal therapies. Counseling around body image issues and sexual health is important for men.

In general, a multidisciplinary approach is used to develop an individualized treatment plan optimal for each male patient. Clinical trials are needed to provide more evidence-based, gender-specific guidelines for men. But the overriding goal remains the same: to provide the most effective curative therapy while minimizing treatment morbidity for men.

Consulting with the Medical Team and Choosing Mastectomy Surgery

After reviewing my options, I decided to undergo a double mastectomy along with reconstructive surgery. Given my cancer characteristics, the medical team agreed this was the best treatment approach.

The tumor was 2 cm and still confined to the breast tissue. But it was Grade 2 aggressive cells with the potential to spread. I tested positive for the BRCA2 mutation, putting me at a high lifetime risk for recurrence.

A lumpectomy with radiation was one option to just remove the tumor. However, the BRCA2 gene mutation made me strongly consider mastectomy for more definitive cancer control.

After much thought, I chose a bilateral mastectomy of both breasts. Removing all breast tissue would lower my risk of the cancer coming back substantially. Though drastic, I felt peace knowing the cancer would be gone for good.

Knowing I would lose an integral part of my manhood was difficult to reconcile. But protecting my health and longevity ultimately outweighed preserving my breasts. I took comfort in knowing reconstruction could aesthetically restore them afterward.

My medical team fully supported my decision. They felt the double mastectomy offered the best long-term outcome, given my circumstances. We scheduled the surgery for a few weeks, allowing time to mentally prepare.

The weeks prior were an emotional rollercoaster. Despite moments of fear and sadness, I focused on the positive. I could move on as a survivor, free from the burden of this diagnosis, once I recovered.

Though the mastectomy felt extreme, I trusted this path would give me the greatest chance to thrive in life after breast cancer.

Preparing Mentally and Physically for an Upcoming Surgery

The weeks leading up to my mastectomy were filled with appointments, tests, and preparations. I wanted to enter surgery in the best physical and mental state possible.

I met with the surgeon to discuss the details of the operation and recovery. He patiently answered my many questions and eased my worries about the procedure.

They did pre-op testing—bloodwork, EKG, chest X-ray, and medical clearance. I got set up with the reconstructive plastic surgeon as well.

At home, I worked on eating well and staying active with exercise. I knew good nutrition and fitness would help my body bounce back stronger.

To build strength for recovery, I walked daily and did light strength training without overexerting myself. I ate a high-protein diet with lots of vegetables and antioxidant foods.

Staying busy and focusing my mind also helped manage anxiety. I made preparations around the house and worked in my absence. I tried to minimize stress where possible in the lead-up.

To prepare emotionally, I leaned on loved ones for support. I also met with a therapist who specializes in cancer patients. She helped me process my feelings about the surgery and hospitalization.

I viewed this journey as both physical and psychological preparation. By taking care of myself, I put myself in the best position to handle surgery and treatment with fortitude.

When the day came to check into the hospital, I felt ready. I was scared but resolute in my decision to go through with it. This marked the beginning of my road to recovery and the new life ahead as a survivor.

Chapter 4

Surgery and Hospital Stay

A Walk-through Mastectomy Surgery Day

The day of my mastectomy surgery finally arrived. I checked into the hospital early in the morning with my wife by my side. After changing into a gown, I was prepped for the operating room.

The nurses started an IV line and went over pre-op protocols. The anesthesiologist then spoke with me about how they would keep me comfortable and pain-free during surgery.

Feeling nervous, I kissed my wife goodbye before they wheeled me off to the OR. The surgical team welcomed me into the cold, sterile room. They reviewed my name and the procedure one last time as they positioned me on the table.

As the anesthesia medications flowed into my IV, I slowly drifted off, the bright surgical lights above me being the last thing I remembered.

The surgeon first performed the mastectomies, meticulously removing all breast tissue down to the pectoral muscles. They sent the tissue for biopsy to ensure clean margins.

Next, the reconstructive plastic surgeon accessed the chest muscle to insert the breast implants that would reshape my chest. After positioning the implants, they closed the incisions.

The lengthy procedure took several hours. I awoke groggy in the post-anesthesia care unit, with quintuple drains sticking out of my bandaged chest. The difficult part was over—my implants had taken the place of my breast tissue. Healing could now begin.

Though still cloudy from anesthesia, I was relieved to have the mastectomy behind me. My wife sat by my side as I dozed in and out, her presence keeping me calm.

One step closer to survivorship, I thought as I drifted off, finally cancer-free.

Hospital Stay and Recovery After Surgery

The first few days after my mastectomy in the hospital were physically and emotionally challenging. I had extensive post-surgical pain and drains to manage. I also grappled with the magnitude of what I had just undergone.

After surgery, I was quite sore and fatigued. The pain medication offered some relief but made me nauseated and dizzy at times. Simple tasks like getting in and out of bed required assistance from nurses.

The drains inserted to prevent fluid buildup were cumbersome. I had to carefully empty and measure the output from each bulb twice daily. I grew accustomed to carrying around the bothersome drains as I started walking the halls.

Early mobility was key to preventing surgical complications like blood clots. But even short, slow walks left me winded. I was anxious to get moving again, but I learned patience while recovering from the invasive surgery.

Mentally, seeing my bandaged, foreign-looking chest was difficult at first. Coming to terms with part of my identity as a man being irrevocably changed took time. Talking through these feelings with a counselor was invaluable.

Overall, I focused on healing—allowing my body time to rest, staying on top of pain control, eating well, and slowly increasing activity. I reminded myself daily that this surgery cured my cancer.

By the time I was discharged home, I felt ready, though still fragile. The hard work of recovering my strength and adapting to life after a mastectomy lay ahead. But the hardest part—saying goodbye to my breasts and the cancer they harbored—was behind me.

Drain Care, Pain Management, and Post-Op Complications

Caring for my post-mastectomy drains was an involved process. I went home with five drains—two per side and one in the center—to prevent fluid from accumulating under my skin.

Twice a day, I had to strip each drain by gently squeezing the tubing. This kept blood and lymph fluid moving through. Then I had to empty and measure the output and record it on a chart.

The bulbs and tubing were cumbersome, but very important to prevent seromas. I made a point to monitor for clogs and keep the sites clean. After a week, as drainage tapered off, the drains were removed.

Managing pain was also crucial for recovery. The prescription medication helped significantly but caused side effects like nausea, fatigue, and constipation. As my pain improved, I transitioned to over-the-counter analgesics.

While inpatient, I was monitored closely for post-op issues like bleeding or infection. Thankfully, I avoided any major complications. However, I did develop superficial cellulitis, which was treated with antibiotics.

Recovering from a double mastectomy was no easy feat. Caring for my drains, keeping pain under control, and healing required diligence. However, any difficulties endured were minor compared to fighting cancer.

I kept perspective by focusing on each small win: walking farther, needing fewer pain meds, and drains coming out. With each step, I grew stronger on my journey back to health as a cancer survivor.

The Art of Resilience During the Difficult Recovery Period

The mastectomy recovery pushed my mental and physical limits. Those first post-op weeks were among the most grueling of my life. But a resilient mindset got me through.

Staying positive was crucial. I focused on my progress each day, not dwelling on discomfort. I reminded myself often that this short-term struggle meant long-term health and survival.

Keeping active also helped tremendously—both exercising and staying busy. Slow, short walks and arm exercises built strength and prevented complications. Gentle stretches kept my limbs loose.

I returned to work part-time after 2 weeks, which helped occupy my mind. Though tiring initially, keeping moving was key. I celebrated each new milestone, like driving again or sleeping comfortably.

Support from friends and family bolstered me during low points. Their visits, meals, and encouragement reminded me I was never alone in this fight. My circle of support kept me going.

Humor played a role too. Even just laughing at funny movies provided an emotional salve when I felt overwhelmed. I refused to lose my ability to smile and laugh, despite the circumstances.

Staying on top of pain control, nutrition, and rest enabled me to rebuild stamina. I listened to my body's limits but progressively increased my activity.

Above all, focusing on the positive implications of the surgery propelled me forward. Each difficult day meant I was getting further from cancer and closer to my healthy future.

My resilience was tested physically and mentally during recovery. But sticking to my survivor mindset got me through the darkest days. If I could overcome mastectomy, I knew I had the inner strength to tackle whatever lay ahead.

Chapter 5

Emotional Impact and Coping Strategies

Struggles with Self-Image After Mastectomy

After the mastectomy, I struggled to come to terms with my altered body and the loss of such an integral male body part. Though necessary, losing my breasts took a heavy psychological toll.

Seeing my chest wrapped in bandages with drains sticking out was difficult. But even after healing, looking at the long, seamed scars across my chest caused sadness and a sense of mourning.

My chest was aesthetically reconstructed to resemble male breasts. But knowing the artificial implants within would never look or feel the same tormented me.

I hid my chest under loose shirts, avoiding my reflection. I dreaded thoughts of baring my scars—either literally in intimacy or metaphorically by sharing my experience.

Despite counseling, I sank into depression as grief over what I lost settled in. I fixated on being "deformed" or "disfigured", fearful of being seen as less of a man.

Friends tried to reassure me that I was alive and cancer-free. My chest did not define my worth. Their masculinity was not destroyed by cancer, so their platitudes rang hollow.

In time, focusing less on what I lost and more on what I gained helped me turn the corner. My perspective shifted from mourning my old chest to appreciating my healthy, strong, cancer-free body.

My journey to rebuild confidence and self-love was a marathon, not a sprint. But coping strategies like counseling, journaling, and support groups gradually moved me from shame to acceptance.

Acceptance was empowering, freeing me to embrace life without inhibitions or limitations because of what I'd overcome.

Coping with Hair Loss, Fatigue, and Physical Changes During Chemotherapy

Despite mentally preparing for it, the physical changes that accompanied chemotherapy were jarring. Losing my hair, stamina, and sense of health during chemotherapy took an emotional toll.

After just a few treatments, my hair started falling out in clumps. Watching my bare scalp emerge in the mirror was upsetting. My thinning hair was a visible, constant reminder of being a cancer patient.

Fatigue also weighed heavily on me, both physically and emotionally. Some days I barely had the energy to get out of bed. Struggling through tasks I once did easily was disheartening.

Appetite changes caused weight and muscle loss that left me feeling weak and feeble. My withering strength and stamina frustrated me deeply.

I was also self-conscious about changes like dry skin or darkened nails. Though minor, they chipped away at my dignity on difficult days.

To cope, I focused on controlling the controllable. I ate nutritious meals even when uninterested in food. Gentle exercise preserves muscle and energy. I stayed hydrated and well-rested.

Wearing hats and headscarves helped me accept my hair loss. I expressed emotions in therapy and in my journal. Spending time outdoors boosted my mood.

Above all, I acknowledged that these changes were temporary means to a permanent end: survival. Keeping my eye on the prize of completing treatment gave me patience and perspective.

While chemotherapy took its toll physically and emotionally, I found healthy outlets to vent, validate, and overcome the difficulties. Using coping strategies was key to preserving my well-being and self-worth.

Seeking Counseling and Peer Support Groups

To help me through the emotional struggles of diagnosis and treatment, I regularly saw a therapist who specialized in counseling cancer patients. She gave me a safe space to process difficult feelings.

In our sessions, I grieved the loss of my former life and health. I vented fears about chemotherapy, death, and the unknown. I expressed stress, anger, and sadness over my reduced independence.

My therapist listened without judgment, validating and normalizing my feelings. She taught me coping techniques for stress and anxiety. Talking about issues left me feeling mentally clearer and less alone.

I also attended a local support group for male cancer patients. Sharing stories and struggles with men who understood what I faced was immensely healing.

We traded practical advice on issues like dealing with hair loss or intimacy after surgery. We discussed current research and treatment options. We laughed together at the absurdities of life with cancer.

My motivation came from the simple fact that I was seen and heard by other survivors who had gone through similar struggles. Their camaraderie normalized situations that others often don't grasp unless personally experienced.

Seeking counseling and peer support were instrumental in safeguarding my mental health. Processing emotions and connecting with those who've been there helped dispel isolation and self-pity.

Working through the psychological impact of cancer strengthened my resilience. I emerged on the other side a more enlightened, empathetic person for having navigated the darkness.

Maintaining Hope and Positivity Throughout My Cancer Treatment

Keeping a positive mindset during the grueling treatments was imperative for persevering through the difficult cancer journey. Though not always easy, hope powered me forward.

I focused on the light at the end of the tunnel—completing treatment and getting back to a normal, cancer-free life. During low moments, I reminded myself that this was temporary.

Celebrating small successes is encouraged—an easy blood draw, a good pathology report, and higher energy levels. Each positive step fueled optimism.

Humor was invaluable, even in dark times. Laughing with loved ones lifted my spirits. Finding the comedy in handling hair loss or donning a hospital gown kept me grounded.

To stave off my fixation on worst-case scenarios, I redirected my mind to gratitude. I focused on what my body could still do, like take short walks or spend time with family.

Faith and prayer offered comfort, helping me surrender my worries. I entrusted my fate to a higher power, releasing what I couldn't control.

Self-care renewed me during the cancer treatment's toll—relaxing baths, soothing music, and comforting foods. Doing little things solely for myself amidst hardship was restorative.

But above all, love powered my spirit when my strength faltered. My family and friends enveloped me in an unbreakable web of support. Their presence gave me courage when mine wavered.

Choosing positivity and hope was a deliberate mindset shift away from despair. Through the worst of times, I managed to stay strong because of my loved ones, humor, and gratitude. And passing through the storm empowered my spirit to shine brighter.

Chapter 6

Life After Cancer

Follow-Up Testing and Surveillance After Active Treatment Ends

After completing surgery, chemotherapy, and radiation, I transitioned into the follow-up phase of care. Though finished with active treatment, I would continue close monitoring.

I saw my oncologist every 3 months for the first year, and then every 6 months after that. At appointments, she examined me for recurring lumps and checked my bloodwork.

I underwent imaging tests periodically to ensure the cancer hadn't returned. Alternating mammograms, ultrasounds, and MRIs revealed my surgical site and remaining tissue.

My doctors also monitored for any secondary cancers. Breast cancer survivors are at higher risk of developing new primary cancers. I was screened regularly for other types.

I educated myself on warning signs like new lumps, bone pain, or breathing issues. Listening to my body and speaking up about any unusual symptoms was imperative between visits.

The surveillance phase can induce anxiety despite being done with treatment. Fear of recurrence is common. I am still tense, awaiting the test results.

But clear scans and bloodwork offer huge relief—reassurance that the cancer remains in the past. My doctor also reassures me that early detection improves outcomes should cancer ever return.

Follow-up care empowers survivors to actively participate in their health. Understanding the monitoring protocol and risks helps alleviate uncertainty.

Through it all, I feel profoundly grateful to be under surveillance rather than active treatment. Moving into long-term follow-up means the worst is behind me as I carefully embrace life after cancer.

My Reflections on Surviving Cancer As a Changed Man

Looking back now as a survivor, I emerge on the other side as a changed man—both emotionally and physically transformed. My scars and story are forever altered by contending with this disease.

The experience endowed me with hard-won wisdom about what truly matters. I see life as precious and fleeting—every day a gift. My priorities shifted away from trivial concerns to cherishing time with loved ones.

I limped through some of the lowest moments a man could face, coming to terms with the loss of my breasts and masculinity. But the crucible empowered me to embrace my new normal, scars and all.

My sense of self-worth no longer hangs on defined pectorals or a full head of hair. Self-love stems from within—how I persevered and overcame.

I waved goodbye to petty vanities, emerging enlightened about sources of meaning. Joy is found in watching my kids grow, feeling sunshine on my face, and living free from tubes and treatments.

Cancer exposed vulnerabilities like mortality and changed looks, burdening many men. But since facing my deepest fears, simpler joys now fill me with wonder.

My hard-won battle has also made me more reverent of the human capacity to heal. With support, our minds and bodies can overcome what seem like insurmountable odds.

While cancer inflicted profound pain, out of the ashes arose growth. I've become more authentic, vulnerable, empathetic, and engaged with life.

My hope in sharing this story is to empower men facing breast cancer to push forward. There is life waiting beyond the struggle. Scars and all, you can survive and thrive as your new best self.

Volunteering to Support Other Male Breast Cancer Patients

After surviving breast cancer, I felt called to give back by supporting other men going through diagnosis and treatment. I began volunteering for cancer organizations, starting support groups, and mentoring newly diagnosed patients.

I provide a listening ear and solidarity for men navigating the challenges I faced not long ago. I offer insights based on my experiences—how I made treatment decisions, stayed mentally resilient, involved family, and more.

I share practical tips on issues important to men that medical teams may overlook: minimizing muscle loss, intimacy after breast surgery, coping with hair loss, and body image changes.

My goal is to help men feel empowered in their fight, knowing someone who's been there is in their corner. I aim to instill realistic hope even in the darkness of a cancer diagnosis.

At support groups, we create a safe space for men to open up about sensitive topics they may not discuss elsewhere. The peer connection provides relief from isolation. Men often feel like rare male "breast cancer patients".

I lobby to raise awareness about male breast cancer, given the lack of public consciousness. Outreach is crucial, so men know to look for symptoms and take them seriously. Early detection saves lives.

Perhaps nothing is more rewarding than mentoring a man from diagnosis through to survival. Journeying with them through treatment's peaks and valleys keeps me motivated.

My cancer experience taught me that coming together to support one another lights the way through our most trying times. Giving back now helps me make sense of the painful odyssey and affirm that I survived not just for myself but to lift others.

Gratitude for Health, Family, and Friends After the Cancer Journey

After the trials of cancer treatment, I emerged with profound gratitude—for my health, family, friends, and the simple joys of life. This hard-won perspective shaped me as a survivor.

My first mammogram after completing treatment delivered the news every survivor longs for no evidence of disease. Reading those words, relief and gratefulness washed over me. I could breathe deeply again; the cancer was truly gone.

I gained immense appreciation for the human capacity to heal during my recovery, both physically and emotionally.

Our resilience amazes me—the way our minds and bodies adapt and overcome illness given time and care.

My family's unwavering support through diagnosis, treatment, and recovery demonstrated true love. I'm so grateful for their strength when mine failed and their laughter that buoyed me. We endured the crucible together, closer than ever.

Good friends became like brothers on this journey, carrying my spirit when I felt too weak to walk. Their encouragement fueled me, and their loyalty humbled me in my most vulnerable moments.

Simply having the opportunity to grow old and watch my children mature is a gift my diagnosis threatened to take away. Every milestone they achieve fills me with joy.

Cancer clarified what matters—not wealth or appearances, but meaningful time with loved ones. My eyes opened to life's beauty amidst hardship.

While cancer inflicted deep wounds, it also revealed light within the darkness. I emerged not unscathed but profoundly grateful for this second chance and the lessons learned about what lasts.

Conclusion

In sharing my personal story of the detection, diagnosis, and treatment of breast cancer as a man, I hope to spotlight key learnings for others facing this disease.

Men, listen to your body and advocate for yourself. Notice any breast changes and push for a prompt diagnosis. Early detection is critical, so speak up about symptoms.

Surgery, while difficult, can save lives in early-stage breast cancer. Consider mastectomy if reducing recurrence risk is a priority.

Recovery takes time and support. Accept limitations post-surgery, but stay as active as possible. Enlist help while building back independence.

Expect a rollercoaster of emotions. Seek counseling to process grief over physical changes like losing your breasts. Peer support provides comfort.

During treatment, focus on what you can control; rest, nutrition, and light exercise. Monitor side effects and get relief. Communicate with your care team regularly.

Life after cancer brings hope but also fear of recurrence. Stay vigilant with follow-up surveillance to enable early re-intervention if needed.

Despite the trauma of cancer, you can survive and thrive. This experience will empower and strengthen you in unimaginable ways.

Breast cancer in men may be rare, but with vigilance and timely treatment, more of us can become long-term survivors. My scars and story stand as a testament that it can be overcome.

By sharing my firsthand account, I aim to raise awareness while reassuring other men facing this battle that they are not alone. Together, through openness, empathy, and courage, we can alter the male breast cancer narrative to one of hope and healing.

A Call to Action for Awareness, Screening, and Support for Men with Breast Cancer

In closing, I issue an urgent call to action to improve awareness, screening, and support for men contending with breast cancer. Though survival rates have improved, more work is needed.

We must educate all men that breast cancer affects more than just women. Promote that men perform regular self-exams and report any breast changes promptly. Earlier stages of diagnosis improve the prognosis.

Press health providers to take breast symptoms in men seriously for timely diagnosis, not downplaying them compared to women. Delays can be devastating.

Encourage high-risk men to pursue supplemental screening like mammograms despite the lack of standard guidelines. Catching cancer early outweighs the risks of extra imaging.

Make counseling and peer support groups more available to help men deal with the emotional impact of breast cancer diagnosis and treatment. Mental health support fosters coping.

Push to include male breast cancer data in research and clinical trials rather than just focusing on women. Gender differences exist; we need male-specific evidence.

Advocate for insurance coverage for wigs, prosthetics, and reconstruction to help offset costs and improve access to these services for men.

But most importantly, speak openly about male breast cancer to chip away at stigma. The more men share their experiences, the more lives can be saved through awareness.

My story is one of thousands, but together, our voices grow louder, supporting and empowering each other. For those newly diagnosed, you are not alone. Together, we can change the future for men facing breast cancer.

Future Outlook and Words of Inspiration

As a survivor several years out, my future outlook shines brightly, unburdened by cancer's grip on me. Though vigilant, I feel hopeful about the road ahead.

Recovery was trying, but I emerged stronger. My hard-won perspective on what matters fuels me daily. I savor a lifetime with family, simple joys, and my health.

To patients newly diagnosed, know that the other side awaits. You will look back as a stronger, wiser version of yourself. Have faith in your resilience.

When fear or sadness overwhelms you, reach out. Your loved ones can absorb the emotions with you, so you don't carry the burden alone.

Focus on each milestone reached, not just the endpoint. Celebrate finishing treatments, clear scans, and days when you feel more like yourself.

On difficult days, nurture your spirit through exercise, nature, and laughter. Release tension through yoga, massage, or counseling. Listen to your mind and body.

You may feel alone as a rare male patient, but an army stands ready to lift you. Support groups connect you to fellow survivors—your band of brothers.

Let vulnerability empower you, not weaken you. Open up about challenges so others can learn how best to support you. Shared struggle builds bonds.

No matter how dark the prognosis is, don't lose sight of hope. Through research and care, breast cancer has become more survivable. You have every reason to believe you will defy the odds too.

Staying positive takes work, but it pays dividends for your health and outlook. Your mindset can be your most powerful weapon to beat this. You've got this!